MAKING
JOINT DECISIONS

ANNE HUNT
Edited by Eric Mein, M.D.

A Note to the Reader

The information in this book is not presented as prescription for the treatment of arthritis. Application of the medical information found in the Edgar Cayce readings and interpreted herein should be undertaken only under the supervision of a physician.

Other Books in This Series

First Printing: March, 1992
Printed in the U.S.A.

For all good and all healing must come from the Divine within each person. As the conscious mind is made aware of the Divine within each cell of the body, there is a greater opportunity for physical applications to result in healing. Based on reading 3512-1

EDGAR CAYCE
PIONEER IN HOLISTIC HEALTH CARE

Table of Contents

PREFACE

It's no secret that our society is in the midst of a health care crisis. The problem is partly economic, as we struggle to find ways to pay for the high level of care made possible by medical technology. It's also a research crisis, as scientists look for cures to diseases such as AIDS. Those are the sorts of problems that make the headlines. Those are the challenges that are clearly evident.

But our health care crisis has more subtle features, too—aspects that are easy to miss but just as important. For example, how much guarantee can doctors give us for our health? How much responsibility are we willing to accept *for ourselves*? Are there some ailments for which *self-care* is not only more economical but also more likely to produce the results we want?

Another elusive feature of our society's health care crisis is in our attitude toward health and healing itself. Recent decades have seen an explosion of alternative health services, many of them claiming to follow a more natural or a more holistic approach.

V

The success of some of these new methods makes us wonder about the validity of the familiar medical model. Is the body really more or less a machine that gets fixed like a balky appliance or a malfunctioning vehicle? Or is the human being a rich, complex mixture of body, mind, and spirit where problems at one level must be addressed at all three?

Working in the first four-and-a-half decades of the twentieth century, Edgar Cayce was a tremendous resource that we can now draw upon to meet the modern crisis in health care. His approach and methods for health maintenance and healing feature self-care that is often, yet not always, in conjunction with a physician's guidance. He was truly a pioneer of the contemporary holistic health movement and ahead of his times in pointing out the attitudinal, emotional, and spiritual components of disease.

Although best known as a "psychic" (or "the sleeping prophet," referring to his occasional predictions about world conditions), Cayce might be better labeled as a "clairvoyant diagnostician" or an "intuitive physician." The point with these descriptive terms is to emphasize first that Cayce's work was principally diagnostic and prescriptive. He was not a healer nor did he have office hours to see patients the way a doctor would. The cases that he took, the people who came to him for help were almost invariably those who had unsuccessfully tried the traditional medical approaches of their day and came to Cayce as a last resort, asking "What's *really* wrong with me? What treatments—no matter how unusual—will bring relief and healing?"

But as descriptive labels for Cayce also emphasize, his method of meeting those requests was intuitive. He had no formal medical school training. Yet he was apparently able to alter his consciousness in such a way that he could see clairvoyantly the real origins of afflictions (physical, mental, and spiritual). What's more, he could then prescribe natural and holistic treatment procedures—sometimes requiring the involvement of a physician or other health care professional, but often needing only a self-care regimen.

The material came through as lengthy discourses (called "readings"), which were stenographically recorded and then transcribed. Most of the information was given for specific individuals and their afflictions, but on occasion there were readings given on particular health topics which contained universally applicable information.

This book is one of a series of volumes in which common ailments and health difficulties are directed. Each topic addresses information given by Cayce which is principally focused upon self-care. The author, Anne Hunt, has carefully researched those readings on the respective health concern, focusing on the treatment procedures that were suggested to many different people as well as those recommendations that were clearly indicated for general use. Her research compilation and writing go a long way toward making these helpful methods accessible to us all. You'll find all the books in this series highly readable and very practical.

Anne's collaborator is Dr. Eric Mein, who served

as medical editor. Sometimes Cayce's language requires the insight of a trained physician to translate concepts into modern terminology. Often there are new findings in medical research that shed light on one of Cayce's ideas. Eric has skillfully added that dimension to the creation of this book.

This particular volume addresses a topic that's familiar to almost all of us: arthritis. Virtually everyone either suffers from this affliction or is close to someone who does. When it hurts simply to move, life can lose a lot of its joy and promise.

Like other Cayce approaches to health, the answer for this problem is a whole body perspective. As much as the discomfort may feel focused in a joint here or there, the *entire body* is involved. What's more—in line with the true spirit of holistic health care—the answer comes from dealing with more than just the physical body. The mind and the spirit play key roles, too. This book will teach you Cayce's physical remedies for arthritis. In addition you'll learn ways to work with your mind (attitudes, emotions, and visualization exercises) and your spirit (ideals, purposes, and meditation) to promote relief from this debilitating disease. The Cayce readings don't claim to have *the* answer to this health dilemma, but they do offer a highly practical, self-care approach to overall prevention as well as treatment.

Mark Thurston, Ph.D.
Association for Research and Enlightenment, Inc.

INTRODUCTION

Central to what defines life is one of its most basic features: the capacity to move. Our ability to transport our bodies through time and space allows us to create and enjoy the world around us—to dance, play with our children and grandchildren, and go for long walks on the beach. We often take this ability for granted until something hampers our movement. Arthritic joint pain can easily affect our capacity to move and do things and hence influences the quality of our lives.

This book contains a unique and holistic approach to the two most common forms of arthritis: osteo- and rheumatoid arthritis. The suggestions found within these pages are based on readings given by Edgar Cayce, one of the foremost psychics of the twentieth century. The majority of his readings dealt with the physical concerns of individuals who sought his advice.

The overall approach of the Cayce source to our bodies involved an intricate living "ecosystem," composed of more than seventy trillion cells, striving together to achieve harmony and health. Like all living systems, these cells were viewed as possessing a robust ability to renew themselves. Far from being passive players in the arthritic process, they were seen as playing a major part in the body's healing forces in its dance back to health. The Cayce readings cited our cells' and bodies' abilities to renew or regenerate as the most fundamental of universal laws applying to our physical system. So health can only emerge as we provide our cells with an optimal environment by meeting their nutritional needs, clearing them of waste products and other toxins, sending them coordinated messages from our nervous systems, and giving them the incentive to renew themselves from our endocrine glands.

The Cayce approach to arthritis emerges from this perspective. Like a garden, our bodies will respond to proper cultivation and nutrients. Such gentle coaxing enables our ecosystem to produce its best fruit, allowing for the enhancement of our entire experience—spiritually, mentally, and physically. While osteoarthritis and rheumatoid arthritis are two different processes, they share many features in common with the readings' approach. The goal of each procedure was initially to cleanse the glandular system (often with the use of Atomidine) to allow for regeneration, and then to work with enhancing the elimination of toxins and the assimilation of the proper nutrients. Heat, Epsom salts, and massage are employed to help stimulate these processes at the joints themselves. Further incentive for healing was given through the Wet-Cell Battery, usually with gold in the solution jar. (These procedures will be clarified in the chapters ahead.)

While some of these therapies are common sense, others are unique to the readings and often difficult to understand and explain. At this time, more work is needed to explore the entire approach, which remains scientifically untested and unproven. Occasionally, however, one encounters hints that there is something to it. For example, when I was reviewing some of the readings given for individuals with osteo-arthritis, the mineral silicon was mentioned in several as playing an important role in the healing process. Unfamiliar with this concept, I scanned numerous nutritional texts and gleaned the following: Until the 1970s, silicon was felt to be a non-essential nutrient. Since then, studies have found that silicon appears to play an important role in the resilience of connective tissue, such as cartilage and bone. This discovery has led to the speculation that silicon is involved in several human disorders, including osteoarthritis. Such types of insights by the readings are exciting and give us incentive to further study their approach.

As you explore these concepts, remember that the bottom line is function—the ability to move and be creative in the three dimensions in which we live. The Cayce readings invite us not only to consider their perspective, but also to test it. Rather than automatically accepting their approach, we are to apply and continue to use those concepts we find helpful. To that end, enjoy this book and work with its suggestions as you continue your journey to health.

Eric Mein, M.D.
Meridian Institute
October, 1991

Chapter 1

SCOPING OUT THE JOINT

KEEP MOVING

A major factor in our happiness as human beings relies in large part upon our ability to go where we want to go—when we want to go. We desire to arrive at our destinations under our own steam and as a result of our own innovation. We have an innate desire to build, to make, to grow, to plant, to design. Though we use our mental and spiritual resources to direct our courses, we carry out our plans with our physical bodies. Part and parcel of our bodies are our joints, the "human hinges" which allow us the movement necessary to simply get things done.

Some of the most challenging undertakings of the human spirit, such as writing a novel or performing brain surgery, cannot be accomplished without the finite movements of the fingers and wrists. Yet, seemingly simple acts, such as getting out of bed in the morning

1

or planting a spring garden, are complex in the number of joint movements required for success. Whether complex or simple, almost everything we do as human beings requires the body to move easily and pain free if the creative process of living is to be enjoyed. Life is full of bending, stretching, twisting, turning, going, coming, and staying. Our joints are key players in the orchestration of our lives.

As millions of individuals will testify, our freedom of movement can be threatened by arthritic pain. When joints are stiff and aching, life can become a burdensome effort. Simple tasks may require painstaking endeavors. More difficult undertakings can slowly but surely seem like impossible dreams. This is the legacy arthritis has been known to leave its victims, young and old. Though injury, birth defects, stroke, and numerous other misfortunes sometimes give rise to physical limitations, arthritis is by far the single greatest crippler which threatens us all.

COMMON FORMS OF ARTHRITIS

The two most common forms of arthritis are osteoarthritis and rheumatoid arthritis. Over thirty-five million people suffer from these diseases to the point that they seek medical treatment. Countless others suffer from the irritation of minor arthritic pain. In fact, almost every adult faces the onset of some osteoarthritic symptoms later in life.

Arthritis is as complex as it is serious. The causes of this potentially crippling disease are no better understood than those of cancer and AIDS—and, though it is not a life-threatening condition, extreme cases can disable and severely limit enjoyment of living. But is there hope? Can the causes of arthritis be uncovered? Its onset prevented? Relief given? A cure found?

The answer to the first question is the most important. Yes. There is hope for any individual seeking to ward off the disease, to help a loved one treat it, or to find relief for one's own existing condition, however painful. The remaining questions regarding cause, prevention, relief, and cure are more illusive. The answers lie within the mysterious workings of the body—a miracle "machine" not fully understood by medical science.

What better resource for understanding the intangible forces within the human body than a man who sought information from an intangible source? Edgar Cayce, long respected as one of the world's most documented psychics as well as the father of holistic medicine, used his psychic vision to diagnose literally thousands of people with common and rare diseases. Of those thousands, hundreds suffered from varying degrees of arthritic pain.

Although Cayce's readings were offered to distinct individuals with varying degrees of symptoms, patterns of causes and therapies surface in his work. These insights provide an individual with a foundation upon which to build a personal plan for prevention and treatment. This book outlines those patterns, explains those therapies, and offers suggestions for one's own individual application of those ideas.

Chapter One through Chapter Four offer general information relevant to those who wish to prevent arthritis as well as to those suffering from osteoarthritis or rheumatoid arthritis. These chapters include general information applicable for both diseases as well as insights on how the body, mind, and spirit can play a role in the prevention and cure of these conditions. Chapter Five describes the most often recommended therapies in the Cayce readings, all brought together as a handy reference guide. And Chapter Six offers specific therapies which will help you or your loved ones begin to take an active role in healing.

As you read along, you'll find Cayce's approach to arthritis to be hopeful and encouraging. First and foremost, it is "drugless"—and primarily involves diet, eliminations, hydrotherapy, spinal manipulation, and massage. Complementing this natural approach is the strong suggestion to incorporate the mind in the healing process—through positive thinking and visualization. This holistic perspective, which has gained Cayce renown and respect, offers a safe and responsible avenue of hope and treatment for arthritis sufferers.

INSIDE THE JOINT

Since arthritis primarily affects the synovial joints and surrounding tissues, it is helpful to understand the basic components of our "human hinges." The synovial joints are encased in a capsule which allows a space between the moving bones. The purpose of these joints is to give us flexibility, mobility, and cushioning. They allow us to move and they absorb the shocks of those movements.

Below are the basic components of your synovial joints and their functions.

Capsule. The joint capsule is composed of two layers: the outer made of fibrous tissue, the inner the synovial membrane. The capsule surrounds the synovial cavity and literally joins the bones. The fibers in the outer layer are often arranged in parallel bundles which can form one type of ligament.

Bones. The skeletal system of the body is composed of bones and cartilage. The bones provide the body with support and protection. Without a skeletal structure, movement would be impossible. Bones also store minerals, principally calcium and phosphorous, that can be relayed to other parts of the body as needed.

Cartilage. Cartilage is the gristle or white elastic connective tissue found at the ends of bones. The presence of cartilage within the synovial joints is important because it allows the bones to move and slide past each other.

Synovial membrane. The synovial membrane, which lines the joint cavity, is made of loose connective tissue, elastic fibers, and fat. It secretes synovial fluid.

Synovial fluid. This fluid performs two very important functions: (1) it provides lubrication so that the joint can move freely and smoothly; and (2) it nourishes the cartilage at the ends of the bones which come together in the joint.

Bursa. Bursa are small sacs located strategically in body tissues to reduce friction between moving body parts. They are designed a bit like joint capsules in that they have an outer casing of fibrous tissue and an inner synovial membrane with a fluid similar to synovial. They are situated among muscles, tendons, ligaments, and the bones to which these tissues are attached.

Muscles and tendons. Skeletal muscle surrounds the joints. These muscles taper off to tendons which attach to the bone at the joint. They provide movement, direction, and support. Many joints rely upon the strength of muscular tissue to prevent dislocation.

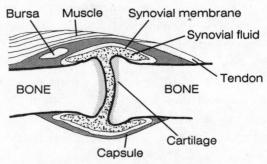

ABOUT OSTEOARTHRITIS

Osteoarthritis is the most common type of arthritis. It affects the lives of almost thirty million people to the degree that they seek out medical treatment. Literally millions of others have a gradual occurrence of the disease in their lifetime. In fact, everyone is likely to have some symptoms of osteoarthritis in varying degrees of severity at some point in time. On one end of the spectrum it can be a minor irritation as the sufferer goes about daily activities. The other end of the spectrum is much more serious, often resulting in disability.

Generally speaking, it is believed that this form of arthritis results from gradual wear and tear of the joints. Thus, it tends to develop with age. It is characterized by softening, flaking, and eroding of the cartilage within the joint capsule. There can be a calcium buildup in the joint, tendons, and ligaments as well. In advanced cases, the bone ends become raw and rub directly against one another. This causes spurs to form at the end of the bone—which are the nodules that appear on arthritic joints.

Osteoarthritis develops gradually and is often undetected, though it may appear to the sufferer to surface suddenly when symptoms become noticeable. Pain and stiffness in the joint areas, especially after activity, are the primary flags of this degenerative disease.

Most often affected are the weight-bearing joints, such as the knees and hips. The fingers and spine are also frequent victims. All other joints can suffer as well, though there is less likelihood of such affliction. One other interesting characteristic of osteoarthritis is that it tends to strike the body in a symmetrical fashion. Thus, if your right hip develops this malady, the left is probably not far behind. These symptoms can begin to appear when individuals are in their forties or fifties, but are most common to an older population. It has been estimated that as much as 30% to 40% of the population age 65 and over have some symptoms which can be attributed to osteo-arthritis.

ABOUT RHEUMATOID ARTHRITIS

Rheumatoid arthritis occurs less frequently. Roughly five million people in this country suffer from its effects. It is by far a more threatening disease than osteoarthritis as it often affects organs of the body as well, though both forms can be debilitating and painful. This type of joint disease literally appears and sometimes disappears with no apparent warning or indication. Even people who struggle with it throughout their lives will find that there are periods when the disease is at its peak—and other often extended times when it lies dormant.

Rheumatoid arthritis is more a disease of the joint tissues characterized by inflammation of the synovial membrane. Bone degeneration, deformity, and dis-ability sometimes result. A myriad of symptoms can herald the unfortunate arrival of this disease, many of which are easily mistaken for flu or other viral infections. Low-grade fever, weight loss, poor appetite, fatigue, depression, and morning stiffness are counted among the warning signs. Hot, swollen, and sore joints eventually reveal the true arthritic nature of this disease.

The joints most often affected by rheumatoid arthritis

are the wrists, knuckles, knees, balls of feet, ankles, and elbows. It usually develops in the third to sixth decade in life, though older persons can fall prey to it as well. It is two to three times more common in women than in men, but in men the disease is more likely to affect organs rather than just the joints.

VISIT YOUR DOCTOR IF . . .

As stated earlier, arthritis is a serious disease with potentially disabling effects. It should be diagnosed as accurately and expediently as possible. Although your interest in this book indicates a desire to take responsibility for your health, a necessary element for treatment of all serious diseases is guidance by a physician, preferably one sensitive to holistic approaches to health care.

Here are the symptoms which should encourage you to seek a professional diagnosis. A joint (including the neck and back) may:

- hurt for more than a month
- appear red or swollen or be warm to the touch
- have been injured in the past
- have increasing pain when bearing weight
- have discomfort associated with other color changes in the limb or any symptoms of weight loss, fever, or night pain

Consider, too, if arthritis runs in your family. If it does, be particularly alert to any one or a combination of these symptoms.

Chapter 2

HEALING MIRACLES CAN HAPPEN

WHERE THERE'S A WILL THERE'S A WAY

This book will give you a substantial amount of practical advice to help you or a loved one prevent, soothe, and treat arthritic pain. But all the advice in the world is only as good as the attitude you hold as you apply the suggestions. Your attitudes and emotions are powerful factors in maintaining good health—and they are frequent culprits when you're ill. In many cases when Cayce gave advice on arthritis, he would instruct the individuals to first adopt a positive mental *and* spiritual attitude before embarking upon any therapeutic regimen. Otherwise, all their efforts would be in vain, he added.

The Cayce readings painted a picture of how your mind relates not only to your body, but to your spirit as well. They indicated time and again that all healing must come from the Divine within each person. This statement was made in dozens of readings, including many of those on arthritis. Cayce went so far as to say that physical therapies, no matter how well conceived and intended, would fall short of the mark if they were not complemented by an understanding of and connection with the Divine. The same is true for any preventative therapy you undertake. You must enlist the wise Healer within to find ultimate health and wholeness.

Here's the way one reading described the connection: "True, physical is physical, mental is mental, and spiritual is spiritual. Yet these are one in their manifestations in the material forces of the body." (1211-2) This simple statement holds the key to health and healing. Inherent in it is the fact that it can be helpful to think of ourselves as having three bodies—a spiritual body, a mental body, and a physical body. All are at work creating the reality of who and what we are as individuals. According to Cayce, there is an inner wisdom in all of us— a wisdom that programs our bodies to function. The source of this wisdom is the Life Force—that mysterious element that breathes life into a being and embraces the essence of that life even after physical death. It is wise beyond even our brightest scientists, our most astute researchers, our most brilliant doctors. Our spiritual bodies are a part of that life force, reflective of its perfection.

But how does it actually relate to and interact

with our physical body? According to Cayce, the endocrine glands are the contact points between our spiritual bodies and our physical bodies. Interestingly, our glandular system plays a vital role in our body's ability to constantly reproduce and regulate itself. We are not static beings born with a certain number of cells that remain alive throughout our lives. We are reproductive beings, constantly re-creating ourselves on the cellular level as cells die and are regenerated. As we discussed before, our joints are kept healthy by this reproductive activity. The wisdom behind the miracle of this self-generation is the Spirit that gives us life.

Since we all draw upon the Life Energy to live and be whole, why is it that we differ so dramatically in our makeup? Why are some of us short, some tall? Why do some of us struggle with poor health, while others seemingly breeze through life with little more than an occasional common cold? Both genetics and our minds build our physical reality. On the one hand, our genetic patterns dictate whether we have a tendency toward better or worse health. In addition, however, Cayce indicated that our minds play a key role in creating our physical health. According to the readings, our mental bodies are half in the spiritual world, half in the physical. A helpful way of thinking about this is to use the analogy of a movie projector. In a sense, it is as though the spirit is like the bright light of the movie projector. Yet it is filtered through the film, which represents our mind and mental patterns. What we view upon the screen is the physical—still composed of light, but filtered through mental patterns.

Our physical bodies are directly affected by these patterns. How we think. The way we view life. Our outlook on daily events. If we are generally positive and constructive in our thinking, we will feel better. If we are loved and love freely, we will have more energy to help others and to help ourselves. Who can testify that this is true? On the other hand, we've all also had down days, thought poorly of an associate, felt that nothing was going right. Energy is almost immediately depleted by such negative thinking, and illness often results. What is happening is that the mind, operating primarily through the autonomic nervous system (where the Cayce readings say our subconscious is housed), is causing short circuits in the messages it is sending to our bodies. When signals are confused, balance within our bodies is disturbed—and balance is necessary for health and wholeness.

THE RIGHT ATTITUDE

You can see the importance of holding a positive, mental attitude that promotes health and healing. Thinking positively helps prevent illness. But when illness is already present, then such thinking helps reduce the possibility of further physical damage from internal stress and opens the physical and mental bodies to the wisdom and healing urges of the spiritual body.

Depending upon the severity of your condition, it will be easier or harder to keep a cheerful outlook about your life and your condition. For some, arthritic pain has had a long-term debilitating effect upon the mind as well as the body. Thus, it is quite understandable that feelings of resentment and depression may have crept in. If you fall into this category, you are not alone. Many others feel the same as you do—and often with just cause. But to get well, you need to try to turn your feelings around. Concentrate on opening your mind to hope. Try to focus on any feeling of improvement in your condition. Begin to visualize health and wholeness. Enlist your mind to help your body. You'll soon learn specific ways to harness your mind to overcome arthritic pain.

But first, give some thought as to *why* you want to be healed.

THE RIGHT PURPOSE

Hand in hand with a positive attitude is the purpose for which you want to be whole and healthy. If your desires for becoming well are totally self-centered, the road may be a long one. A central idea in the Cayce readings is that we are here on earth to be companions with fellow humans and with God, and as such we must all seek to be of service to one another. Our bodies are not only the sacred temples for our souls, they are also the instruments by which we can serve one another and God. Cayce gave the following eloquent prayer to one arthritic, asking that he use it, in his own words, every day as he went about the healing process:

Our Father who art in heaven, hallowed by Thy name! May the love, O God, Thou has shown to the sons of men, be manifested in me and my body in such measures that I may show forth to my fellow men Thy love as is manifested through the gift of Thy Son to those who have lost their way. May my body, my mind, be used in a service to Thee, through the kindnesses, the gentlenesses, those hopes that may be brought to my fellow men by and through the efforts of my body, my mind, my activities; that all the glory may be to Thee. In His name we seek, O God! (1211-2)

A prayer such as this can have a positive effect upon all your efforts. Incorporate one into your quiet time and it will build positive energy to help you bring about healing.

ALIGN WITH THE SPIRIT

It becomes evident when studying Cayce's philosophy that alignment with the spirit is the key to physical healing. "Do not begin the physical applications until the spiritual body has been renewed. " (3512-1) But how does one renew the spiritual body? Meditation and prayer are key tools to help make this alignment.

Meditation, which may seem like an odd preventative therapy for arthritis, is the act of quieting and emptying oneself so that God's love can be felt, so that His message can be heard. Through

15

prayer, we speak to God with our feelings and thoughts and often ask Him for direction. Then we listen. This act of listening on an inner level is a key ingredient in meditation. When we do so, we become more and more receptive to the Divine Healer within.

QUIET TIME

Here are the key elements that are important in meditation. You may be surprised at how simple they are. Practice them with consistency, and you'll soon begin to feel the results.

Set a Regular Time As you have probably learned in your own life, human beings are creatures of habit. Setting a regular time for any activity, whether it be an evening walk or a morning break, makes it much more likely that you will indeed undertake that activity. Meditation is no exception. If you set a regular time for meditation, perhaps fifteen to twenty minutes for starters, you will find it easier to actually devote time to this important process. Also, you will discover that settling into the routine of meditation allows you to quiet and focus your thoughts more readily. It is as though your mind gets in the habit of a quiet time and thus slips into the meditative state with greater ease.

Learn to Relax If you could learn to relax on a regular basis, your overall health would improve immeasurably. One of the simplest benefits of regular meditation is that you find a small amount of time daily to relax body, mind, and soul. Believe it or not, no matter how hectic may be the day which looms ahead or spirals behind, relaxation can be yours with relative ease.

Here are some powerful relaxers to consider:

Light stretching. Just prior to meditation take a moment to stretch your body by simply reaching upward, straightening your spine. Do whatever stretching motions feel good to you, noticing the release of tension in your muscles.

Head and neck exercise. A specific exercise which is especially helpful prior to meditation is the head and neck exercise, which is described in detail on page 49. This exercise releases tension and increases circulation to the head and neck area.

Soothing music. Gentle music can provide a special nourishment to the soul. Playing peaceful and calming music in the background during meditation can help your mind release the cares of the day and thus focus more adeptly during the meditative process.

Reading inspirational or spiritual verse. Another quieting activity is to select a special book, perhaps the Bible or a favorite book of poetry, to read for a moment as you settle down to meditate. Let your mind focus on the positive images and thoughts as you read.

Breathing. Special breathing techniques can be a tremendous relaxation aid. Here's a simple one with which to begin. As you relax, inhale deeply, visualizing peace and calm flowing in. Then breathe out deeply, releasing any tension and stress you might have as you exhale. Continue this technique until you begin to feel more tranquil.

Sit or Lie with Your Spine Straight It is important during meditation to assume a position with your spine as straight as possible. This allows for the best flow of energy throughout your body. You may choose to sit in a straight-backed chair or in the lotus position, or even lie flat on your back. If you are sitting, place your hands, open and relaxed, in your lap. If you are lying on your back, join your hands over your abdominal area.

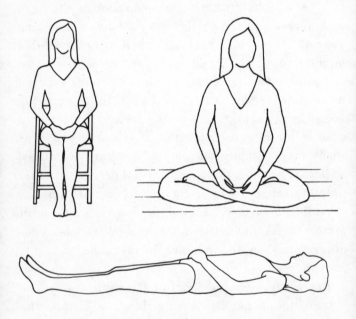

Begin with Prayer Begin your meditation time with a few moments of prayer. In your prayer, remember to be open to God's will, as in the prayer given on page 15. During this time, try to establish a sense of peace and calm within yourself as well as a sense of openness and willingness to be of service. Once you have quieted yourself, it is time to begin meditating.

A special note is important here. If you are unable to become peaceful within, perhaps because you are anxious or upset about something in your life, remain in a prayerful state. Attempting to meditate while feeling negative emotions can stir up those feelings to an even greater extent. Wait until you are in a more congenial mood and later try to meditate again.

Work with a Special Affirmation An affirmation or inspirational phrase is an important element of meditation. It may be a version of the prayer from the Cayce reading mentioned earlier in the discussion about purposes. It might be a brief quotation from the Bible that provides you with inspiration or a short verse you write yourself. Whatever phrase you choose, the essence of it should encompass your highest ideals and principles. Use this phrase as a focal point for your experience. You will probably want to change your affirmation from time to time. It is wise, however, to use the same one for a week or two at a time, so that you become familiar with it. Just like selecting a specific time for meditation, using a familiar affirmation helps make your meditation period more successful. We are, after all, better at what we practice!

Experience the Silence Following your time of silent prayer, begin to repeat your affirmation softly.

Try to focus on and experience the *meaning* or *spirit* of the words. The feelings your affirmation creates should begin to make you experience an upliftment and a greater peace. When you sense that you have raised your consciousness above your ordinary state, become quiet and focus upon that feeling or spirit which the affirmation has created. Hold this spirit for as long as you are able.

Deal Positively with Distractions It is quite natural to get distracted by other thoughts as you meditate. When this occurs, do not become discouraged and quit. Ask for a blessing upon whatever has distracted you and begin to repeat your affirmation. You may choose to simply think about the words of the affirmation at this point, rather than speaking them aloud. Once you have recaptured their spirit and feel more elevated, stop thinking about the specific words once again. Simply focus upon the inner silence you have created. This inner silence is the essence of meditation. In this silence you encounter the spirit, love, and wisdom of God.

Close with a Prayer for Others During meditation you have tapped into a spiritual energy which needs to be dispersed as you conclude this time period. Do so by ending your meditation period with a prayer for others. This selfless act will complete your quiet time in a positive way.

SUMMING UP MEDITATION

Meditation and prayer are vital ingredients in the Cayce readings' approach to illness. Don't be concerned about having a particular kind of experience while you're meditating. Although it's possible that you'll feel the healing energies as you meditate, many people don't directly experience what's actually going on at the subtle levels of their bodies and minds. Don't worry if you don't have a mystical experience. Be assured that positive changes are going on beneath the surface. Through this kind of attunement to the Spirit, Cayce indicated that therapies applied "externally, internally, through the diet, through all portions of the activities, may bring coordination, cooperation in the physical forces of the body. " (1211-2) So, take the time to meditate. It will be an important element in your journey toward recovery.

POWER OF THE SUBCONSCIOUS MIND

The subconscious mind is a powerful ally in your quest for healing and new-found wholeness. As we discussed earlier, this level of the mind directs much of the activity of the autonomic nervous system, which is sending signals to the farthest outposts of your body—signals which can either bring health or illness. Meditation will help you align your mental and spiritual bodies with the Spirit. Pre-sleep suggestions and visualization will be further aids in materializing the wisdom of the Spirit, through the mind, into the body, into the joints.

PRE-SLEEP SUGGESTIONS

The Cayce readings recommended a powerful, useful, and effective method for implanting positive, constructive thoughts in the subconscious to help bring about beneficial change. The readings indicated that the subconscious mind is very accessible and open to suggestion just prior to the time one goes to sleep. So the use of these "pre-sleep" suggestions can gently persuade your mind to construct a foundation of positive thoughts upon which to build your new life style.

To harness the power of these thoughts to help overcome arthritis, you'll want to make your own pre-sleep tape. Making this tape is actually quite easy. Begin by reading through the following script to become familiar with it. Feel free to modify it to make it more personalized for you. Follow only one rule in doing these minor changes—make sure that any words or phrases you substitute will be positive and uplifting. Once you are comfortable with your script, sit down with a tape recorder and record, using a soothing, slowly paced voice and pausing comfortably between phrases (indicated by " . . . "). You might like to have soothing music playing in the background so that it is a backdrop to your voice. This tape of affirmations will help you program your subconscious to develop positive mental attitudes and patterns about healing.

You will gain the optimum benefit from this tape by listening to it on a nightly basis just as you are going to sleep. For best results play the tape at a soothing and comfortable volume near your bedside. If you have a continuous-play cassette recorder that will play both sides of a tape consecutively, you may want to record the script on each side of the tape so that it can play twice as long without interruption. Most important, set the tape up so that it turns off automatically.

PRE-SLEEP TAPE SCRIPT

"Allow your eyes to close now . . . to rest and relax and feel the peacefulness of sleeping . . . focus on your breathing, notice how more peace comes with every breath . . . and deeper relaxation . . . feel the relaxation that your rhythmic breathing brings to your body . . . with each breath, you relax more and more . . . breathe in . . . and out . . . and in . . . and out . . . notice how you are more and more relaxed . . . you are opening to new ways of seeing your life . . . your mind is opening to the healing of the Spirit . . . you can feel the soothing waves of the Spirit . . . you are open to healing . . . to the healing of the Spirit that is a part of you . . . you are feeling relaxed now . . . your body is at peace . . . and it is comfortable and resting . . . your spirit is soothing your body and your mind . . . you are a whole and harmonious being . . . you are beginning to feel lighter, your body feels looser . . . you are ready to allow your body to heal itself . . . to allow its wisdom to bring it harmony and balance . . . you are helping your body heal itself . . . you are friends with your body . . . you love your body . . . you want to help it receive the healing energy of your spirit . . . you know that it can be healed . . . your body can be healed . . . you are giving your body what it needs to be healed . . . you are eating good foods for your body . . . foods that bring a gift of healing . . . foods that bring health and healing . . . you enjoy these foods . . . see how they are making you stronger . . . and more flexible . . . they are soothing your body . . . and giving it nourishment to heal itself . . . your body is becoming happier and stronger and more optimistic . . . you and your body are open to the healing gifts of the foods you eat . . . allowing them to regulate your body in all that it does each day to help you feel better . . . your body is your friend and it is helping you feel better . . . it is drawing on the Spirit to heal itself and help you feel better . . . stronger . . . more flexible . . . more flexible . . . feel how relaxed your body is as it goes about this natural healing process . . . floating into your mind is a vision of your body whole and perfect . . . the way it was created . . . you are moving in the vision gracefully and with vitality . . . your body is healed . . . and radiates the light of the Spirit within . . . your body is radiating the light of the Spirit within . . . you see yourself helping others . . . serving others . . . you are seeing the ways that you want to help and serve others . . . in your vision you are helping others . . . see how good you feel . . . knowing that you are using your body to help others . . . to be of service to others . . . allow your mind to paint a picture of yourself helping others . . . see how this vision of helping others can live in your mind . . . feel how it becomes a seed planted in your mind . . . as it grows . . . your body finds it easier to heal itself . . . easier to listen to the healing whisperings of your spirit . . . your seed of helpfulness to others is growing with time . . . see how it is growing into a tree with many branches . . . see how the seed is growing . . . the branches giving it beauty . . . and spreading out to touch others . . . to offer shade and comfort to others . . . you are like this tree . . . growing stronger . . . helping others more and more as you heal . . . this tree is like your body . . . growing so that it can be of service to others . . . plant this vision, like a seed, in your mind and watch it grow . . . water it with love and nourishment . . . water this vision with love and nourishment . . , giving your body what it needs to be a part of this vision . . . you love your body . . . and your mind is full of love . . . and your spirit is whispering to you secrets of healing . . . and you are listening . . . and you are hearing . . . and you are listening . . . and you are hearing . . . and the Spirit is healing you . . . the Spirit is healing you . . . you are drifting into a natural, comfortable sleep . . . a place where you are safe and at peace . . . you are being carried into sleep as if on gentle rolling waves . . . waves that caress your body . . . your feelings . . . and your soul . . . you hear your inner Spirit . . . whispering to you the secrets of healing . . . your body is being bathed in these whisperings . . . it feels good to you . . . your body is your friend . . . and you are happy that you can help it be healed . . . '

VISUALIZATION

Visualization can be used in a very specific way to help bring about healing of particular joints. In one reading, Cayce told a woman to study not only the anatomy of her condition but the chemistry of it as well. Then, he instructed her to visualize the necessary forces which would bring about healing. This advice points out once again the importance of understanding your ailment, through discussion

25

with your physician or therapist and your own personal research. Know what you hope to accomplish by your therapies. Then, visualize success.

You can improve the effectiveness of your visualization efforts if you go to your local library and spend some time with a good anatomy book. Take note of the structure of your joints, the fascinating descriptions of how your elimination systems work, and the diagram of your spine and nervous systems. Read about the functions of your glands. Most important, look at the pictures! See how your body is constructed. This effort will help you use more effectively the visualization suggestions which accompany the therapies in Chapter Five to bring about healing.

Another way to use this technique is to visualize the nutrients from the foods you eat being assimilated and distributed to all areas of your body, especially to your joints. Picture the energy which the foods you eat provides. As you drink water and eat fiber, see the cleansing effect these substances have upon your body. As you work with this visualization suggestion regarding diet, you'll begin to devise some variations of your own. You'll be amazed at the results.

Basically, these visualization exercises work in the same way that pre-sleep suggestion works. You're helping your subconscious mind, which is closely aligned with your autonomic nervous system, to bring about the changes you hope to accomplish. Visualization can help break down barriers within your mind which may have hindered previous attempts at healing.

MIND OVER MATTER

Now that you've learned how to put "mind over matter," you're ready to learn a bit more about the physiological aspects of arthritis. You've learned that hope lies within your spirit, for your spirit is the key to your healing. But, as Cayce said, it's important to complement your spiritual and mental work with an understanding of how your body works. Now, it's time to look at the causes, preventative measures, and therapies for the healing of arthritis.

Chapter 3

CAN CAUSE LEAD TO CURE?

A MYRIAD OF CAUSES

Many causes behind these joint problems have been considered, researched, and explored. Among them are an abnormality of the immune system or the presence of an infectious agent (for rheumatoid arthritis) to an unstable balance of calcium in the body or simple wear and tear of the joints (in the case of osteoarthritis). Research even points to allergies as playing a role in the creation of some forms of arthritis. All of these imply that this disease can be the result of some form of systemic disorder—a disorder that is universal to the body rather than specific to the joint.

Years before medical science focused on these potential causes of arthritis, Cayce himself was viewing the disease as a manifestation of a larger problem within the complex system of an individual's body.

CAYCE ON CAUSES

In regard to arthritis Cayce identified many causes which are both unique *and* at the same time seem to have a correlation with current research findings. Although we've noted that the readings were always given to individuals with specific symptoms and histories, the following possible causes offer insights potentially helpful to any individual suffering with joint disease.

Here's a list of the most frequently mentioned origins of arthritic problems, common to both osteoarthritis and rheumatoid arthritis:

- poor elimination
- poor assimilation of nutrients
- glandular disorder
- chemical imbalance
- pressure in the cerebrospinal system

All of the above conditions have an adverse effect upon the natural balances within the body and interfere with its ability to maintain and restore health. They can cause toxic buildup, vitamin and mineral deficiencies and overabundances, misdirected metabolic functions, and numerous other conditions which are detrimental to one's general health. The result? A disturbance in the "climate" necessary for a smoothly operating joint.

POOR ELIMINATIONS

The body's major elimination systems are the kidneys, colon, liver, skin, and lungs. If any or all of these organs are not functioning properly, your body will experience a toxic buildup in the blood, lymph, and tissues. This buildup can cause the body to go into overdrive to try to rid itself of these toxins. The result is less regenerative energy in the joints and surrounding tissues. Your body is literally diverting life-giving energy to try to balance out the eliminations. Thus, as cells in tissue, bone, and cartilage die, they may not be replaced by healthy, properly functioning ones. Also, when the eliminations are disturbed, your absorption of nutrients is often hampered, once again making it difficult for your body to regenerate itself. Your general health and well-being then become at risk.

POOR ASSIMILATION

Mentioned briefly above, assimilation is a bodily process of which many people are unaware. We tend to feel that if we eat right, our bodies get the right nutrition. This, however, is not entirely true. Diet, nutrition, and assimilation are not synonymous terms. Here's a much better way of defining these processes. Diet is simply what you eat. Thus, a banana is a part of your *diet*. Its *nutritive value* includes many vitamins and minerals, potassium being a significant mineral and vitamin C an important vitamin. Whether or not the nutritive value of a banana is *assimilated* depends upon many factors, including what other foods are eaten with it, the state of your elimination system, and the condition of your body's glandular system. Whatever the cause of poor assimilation, the result is the same. Lack of proper nutrition intake robs your system of what it needs to function correctly. The vital energies needed to direct your body's varied activities begin to be in short supply. Every corner of your body can suffer, your joints included.

GLANDULAR DISORDERS

In the readings glandular imbalance was one of the most frequently mentioned causes of rheumatoid arthritis. The glands play a vital and often underestimated role in physical health. The term *gland* has a very broad meaning. It refers to any cell or group of cells that secrete substances which help regulate the body's activity. While the endocrine glands secrete hormones, other glands such as the liver secrete substances which are also involved in the body's metabolic processes.

Specifically, Cayce mentioned the thyroid and the adrenals as being involved in the onset of rheumatoid arthritis. An imbalance between the kidneys and the liver, especially as related to their role in handling eliminations, also received special notice. Other references to the glands and glandular forces were more general in nature.

The bottom line would seem to be, however, that an imbalance of the glandular system could result in poor performance of the eliminating organs, poor assimilation of nutrients, a chemical imbalance of different nutrients, and numerous other systemic disorders which could contribute to arthritic conditions.

CHEMICAL IMBALANCE

A chemical imbalance within your body can be the result of poorly functioning glands, poor assimilation, problems with eliminations, erratic nerve impulses, and numerous other sources. In the case of osteoarthritis, the readings referred to the mineral silicon as playing a role in the disease process. Also, Cayce therapeutically recommended iodine in the system as a way to help improve glandular function. The delicate balance of chemicals in your body is necessary for the health of every individual cell. As discussed before, every cell within every joint is vital to the overall well-being of tissue, bone, and cartilage.

PRESSURES IN THE CEREBROSPINAL SYSTEM

Your spine could easily be named the central communications network of your body. Nerve impulses move through your spine, directing your body's complex activities. Any disruption can affect many vital activities. One common source of altering the balance of nerve communications is the improper movement or positioning of a vertebra, sometimes called a spinal lesion or subluxation by the readings. In the case of osteoarthritis, Cayce often pinpointed the lower part of the spine as a problem area. Interrupted or excessive spinal impulses can disturb the life and healing forces of your body. Eliminations can be disturbed, assimilation hindered, glandular activity made erratic.

The results may be a compendium of the health-threatening conditions discussed earlier. Your joints can suffer by becoming a repository of toxic substances, cells can degenerate due to lack of nutrition and energy, and arthritic conditions can set in to the weakened and debilitated areas.

CIRCLE OF HEALTH

As you read about the possible causes of arthritis, you no doubt recognize that they are interrelated. Viewed from a negative angle, this interrelatedness could appear to be a vicious circle, of which it may be difficult to break out. But from a positive perspective, the picture is of a harmonious circle of health, where body systems help each other find balance. Hand in hand, these systems create the miracle of the human body, designed for perfect health.

Chapter 4

ARTHRITIS PREVENTION PLAN

YES! PREVENTION IS POSSIBLE

Now that you know the possible causes of arthritis you can work to prevent it! Prevention is, after all, the best cure for any health problem. The way to keep from succumbing to a disease is to maintain a balance within the body, which in this case would ward off the onset of arthritis.

Thus, the wise course to prevention is to:
- eat right
- keep your eliminations functioning properly
- stimulate proper balance of your glandular system
- promote optimum assimilation of nutrients
- maintain healthy circulation
- preserve spinal health
- think positively!!!

All of these prevention tips are interrelated. Proper eliminations and a properly functioning glandular system promote assimilation of nutrients. Good circulation is a key to optimum delivery of nutrients and removal of wastes. An aligned spine insures that nerve impulses directing your body's activities are balanced. Again, it's the circle of health where systems aid one another in their complex tasks.

EATING RIGHT

The following basic health guidelines are powerful preventers of arthritic disease. Cayce suggested that general health is promoted by a diet which is alkaline in nature. He reiterated this approach to diet to those suffering with arthritic disease and gave one important helpful hint: that the proper diet to help correct this disease is one which is laxative in nature. Vegetables should be the cornerstone of this diet. You'll see below that they are an important ingredient in the Cayce dietary information.

The following guidelines are excellent for prevention *and* they form the backbone of the more specific diet arthritics should follow (described in Chapter Six).

BASIC DIET GUIDELINES

Alkaline-Forming Foods
(Optimally 80% of Your Diet)

All fruits except cranberries, plums, and prunes

All vegetables except for lentils and corn

All milk, including buttermilk

Almonds, brazil nuts, chestnuts, coconut, hazelnuts

Coffee, tea, molasses, brown sugar, brewer's yeast

Acid-Forming Foods
(Optimally 20% of Your Diet)

All meats except for mincemeat

All cereals and bakery products except for soybeans

All cheeses and eggs

Peanuts, pecans, walnuts

WISE COMBINATIONS

The following combinations of foods were suggested by Cayce as being particularly beneficial:

At least three vegetables that grow above the ground for each that grows below the gound

Gelatin with fruits and vegetables to help absorb nutrients

Figs, dates, and corn meal

Small amounts of lemon or lime juice with orange or grapefruit juices

The following were mentioned as being detrimental to your general health:

Milk at the same meal with citrus fruit and juices

Cereals at the same meal with citrus fruits and juices

Coffee with milk or cream

Raw apples eaten at the same time as other foods

Two or more starches at the same meal
Sugary foods with starches
Meats and cheeses with starches

WATER OF LIFE

An important supplement to the above diet is
the proper intake of water. Put simply and with little
fanfare, drink six to eight glasses of water a day.
Intake of an adequate amount of water benefits all
your elimination systems. Here's a suggested routine
which will help you get into the healthy habit of
drinking enough water daily. This routine adds up
to an intake of eight-and-a-half glasses, thus giving
you some cushion in case you miss a glass or two
(but not more) during the day. Notice that the first
half glass of water in the morning is warm. Cayce
suggested this specifically as an aid to help the
digestive system work its best.

When	Count
Upon arising (warm)	1/2
Mid-morning and afternoon	2
Before breakfast, lunch, and dinner	3
After breakfast, lunch, and dinner	3
Total	8 1/2

GELATIN

Here's an unusual tip for assisting your body in
the assimilation of nutrients. The recommendation

was to include unflavored, natural gelatin in your raw vegetable or fruit salad to aid your body in the absorption of nutrients, especially vitamins. What makes this work? It's simple. Gelatin acts as an enzyme in the body, which assists in digestion and the routing of nutrients. So, take this simple advice. Purchase pure gelatin at your grocery store, put it in a salt shaker, and add it to your fruit juice, or prepare congealed vegetable and fruit salads. One specific recommendation for rheumatoid arthritis in the readings was to make a gelatin salad from celery, carrots, lettuce, and watercress. It was indicated that these foods would build the nerve forces within the body, thus bringing about greater health. Gelatin is a tasteless, powerful medicine you'll find easy to take.

JERUSALEM ARTICHOKES

Jerusalem artichokes are new to many people but are actually a very common root vegetable. Little, potato-like tubers of the sunflower family with small blooms and coarse leaves, they have an enjoyable flavor and a crisp texture much like water chestnuts. While Cayce did not specifically suggest these for arthritis, he recommended that some individuals eat one small Jerusalem artichoke three times a week. The first should be eaten raw, the second steamed, the third raw.

Does this root vegetable seem like an odd recommendation for any diet? According to Cayce, the artichoke is a source of natural insulin and would help stimulate eliminations and aid general circulation. Both of these benefits assist your body in toxic cleanup. Include these crispy treats in your diet if you have reason to believe you have need for these benefits.

BEEF JUICE

Beef juice helps build the blood without introducing excess amounts of fat into the system. In several readings, especially when the individual was debilitated, Cayce suggested that the diet be blood building, as iron is a necessary mineral for bodily strength and energy. Preparation of beef juice is really very simple. To begin, gather these items:

1/4 lb. of raw, lean beef
One 32-oz. empty glass jar with top
Large sauce pan
Small wash cloth

Place wash cloth in bottom of sauce pan (this will prevent jar from breaking or cracking). Remove fat from edges of beef and cut the beef into 1-inch cubes. Place these in jar. Cover with top very loosely. Place jar on top of cloth in pan. Fill sauce pan with enough water to come half-way up side of glass jar. Bring water to a boil. Then, simmer for two to three hours, adding water to pan as necessary.

When done, remove from heat and let jar and contents cool. Then, squeeze excess juice from meat into the jar. Discard meat. Refrigerate the liquid. Take not more than a tablespoonful two to four times a day, sipping it *very slowly*. Do not keep the juice longer than three days in the refrigerator.

MUMMY FOOD

Another blood-building food recommended in the readings has a rather strange name: Mummy Food. The origin of this name comes from a dream of Edgar Cayce's in which an Egyptian mummy actually gave him the recipe for this cereal. But don't let the name fool you into thinking that this food tastes stale and musty. On the contrary, it is rich in several minerals necessary for a healthy body and is naturally sweet and tasty. Of course, figs and dates are natural laxatives, which Cayce indicated are good for those suffering with arthritis.

Here's a simple recipe for Mummy Food, which you can prepare as a hot cereal. Begin by gathering the following ingredients:

1 cup black figs
1 cup dates
1/2 cup coarse yellow corn meal
2 1/2 cups of water

Finely chop figs and dates either with a knife or in a food processor or blender. Add the corn meal. Place mixture in a pan with water and cook over low to medium heat for 10—20 minutes, stirring frequently. Heat until cereal is of desired consistency, feeling free to adjust amount of water to your particular tastes.

Serve hot and with milk if desired.

TYPICAL MENU

The following menu gives you an idea of the general approach you should take to your diet. Three meals a day is an important part of the food formula—helping your body maintain a regular level of nutritional intake. Cayce prefaced this menu with a statement indicating that it is simply a guideline to be considered. There are dozens of variations within these suggestions, allowing you to enjoy a diverse and interesting diet.

Mornings. Have either a dry, high-fiber cereal, a hot grain cereal, or citrus fruit whole or as juice. If you enjoy toast, dark bread toast such as pumpernickel, rye or whole wheat is best. You may have a moderate amount of coffee but Cayce warned against having cream in it, indicating that this combination was a stress upon the heart and the digestive system.

Noon. Raw vegetables, as fresh as possible—especially carrots, celery, lettuce, and any other green vegetable. Vegetable soup is a good option for a cold day. Pure, fresh carrot juice, even in as small a quantity as an ounce, is an excellent supplement to this meal. A slice or two of whole wheat bread rounds out your noon meal with added nutritive value.

Dinner. A little meat, if desired, preferably fish, fowl, and lamb. Include shellfish—high in iodine content and thus good for your thyroid. Include an abundance of cooked vegetables, eliminating potatoes. Yams can be enjoyed occasionally.

CLEAN UP YOUR ACT

The food you eat is only as good as your ability to assimilate its nutritive value. Your digestive organs play a vital role both in this process and with eliminations. Thus, keeping your eliminations in tiptop shape helps these organs function and is a vital strategy for insuring proper assimilation. It's wise to understand your body's elimination processes and what you can consciously do to assist them in their mission.

The body's major elimination systems—the kidneys, colon, liver, skin, and lungs—are key players in this strategy. If they are not properly functioning, a toxic buildup in your system results. In turn, your body spends vital energy trying to deal with the excess wastes, depleting the energies necessary for proper assimilation.

Your body is called upon to dispose of many different kinds of waste on a daily basis. For example, there are, of course, the byproducts of what you eat—including the additives and preservatives plentiful in many of today's foods. Also, there are the pollutants you take into your system through your lungs, not to mention chemicals you often unknowingly take in through your skin. Compound these with internally generated wastes: energy that is burned creates waste byproducts, and—believe it or not—billions of cells die each day. All these must be removed from your body to allow for an optimum level of assimilation.

Here's an outline of your body's elimination systems and therapeutic suggestions for keeping them in order.

DYNAMIC DUO

According to the Cayce readings, the kidneys actually function in an equal partnership with the liver. Both process the blood, filtering it for wastes and preparing those wastes for disposal. Any imbalance between these two organs can overwork one and risk the possibility of toxins being thrown back into the system. The best routine to follow to keep the kidneys and liver healthy and effective is to drink six to eight glasses of pure (preferably spring) water a day. A routine for the intake of this amount of water was given earlier.

COLON HEALTH

Besides consuming an ample supply of water each day, make certain to include a substantial amount of fiber in your diet. The diet outlined earlier is high in fiber content. Be sure to include in this diet natural laxatives, such as figs and raisins, and your colon will reap the benefits. An occasional colonic by a professional therapist or a self-administered enema will also be of benefit. A periodic internal cleansing of the colon makes sense. No matter how fibrous your diet or how consistent you are in your intake of water, there will be a buildup of wastes clinging to the walls and hiding in the folds of the colon. An internal cleansing with water and a mild antiseptic will help keep your colon functioning at its optimum level.

What if you can't find a colonic therapist? Then administer an enema to yourself at home. Though a colonic is as effective as four to six enemas—say the readings—an internal cleansing of either kind, carefully administered, will have tremendous effects on your health. See Chapter Five for directions on administering an enema.

There's also a special Cayce readings' therapy which is recommended to stimulate the liver, gall bladder, and colon. It is one of the most unique therapies suggested in the readings: the castor oil pack. The use of this pack, applied externally, was recommended literally hundreds of times. Chapter Five offers directions for applying this pack.

LUNG POWER

As your body burns energy, it converts your oxygen intake to carbon dioxide which must be expelled through the lungs. Fresh air and deep breathing are the cornerstone of healthy eliminations through the lungs. All the exercises described later in this chapter, especially the "Morning Wake-Up," will help stimulate toxic release through the lungs. In general, remember to get as much fresh air as possible, breathing deeply and exhaling forcefully. Breathing is one of our most important bodily functions (obviously!) and yet goes with little notice and less genuine care. Simply paying attention to your breathing patterns and affording yourself the regular opportunity for fresh air will have a positive effect on your health.

YOUR SKIN AT WORK

Perspiration is an important process in general and is particularly beneficial to another of your body's elimination organs: the skin. Any exercise or activity you engage in that produces perspiration is doing your elimination systems a world of good. Every drop of water leaving your body carries toxic wastes.

Another way of increasing perspiration is to take a steam bath. The best route for obtaining a steam bath is in a health facility that provides this service. Many massage therapists, for instance, will have a steam cabinet available for you to take a steam before your massage. Also, you may belong to a health club with a steam room. If you do, don't overlook the benefit of a good five- to ten-minute steam.

But steams aren't relegated to only the fortunate few who have access to such facilities. Hydrotherapy can also be administered at home. See Chapter Five for directions on giving yourself a home steam.

KEEP MOVING

Cayce was an advocate of moderate, regular exercise to stimulate circulation. Stretching was recommended time and again as being beneficial to the body. Walking was mentioned as an exercise which would be good for anyone. Swimming and rowing were two water sports that got favorable reviews as well by Cayce's psychic source. When you choose your exercises and sports, do those which are easy on the joints.

Traumatizing your joints can make your arthritis worse. The more well-rounded your exercise program, the more enjoyable and beneficial it will be.

Here's a general principle you can use in designing your exercise routine. In the mornings exercise the upper portion of your body. This will help bring your blood to the upper body—and to your head so that you can start thinking clearly before beginning your daily routine. So, if you take a morning walk, swing your arms as you go along. This will cause your body to pump blood to the upper extremities.

In the evenings do just the opposite. Exercise your lower body to help draw blood from your head and neck and increase trunk circulation—thus promoting much needed relaxation after a long day's activity. This enhances body-building functions as well.

Exercise stimulates circulation and glandular activity. It gets the heart pumping, the blood and lymph flowing. As your lungs expand and contract in exercise, toxins are released. Last but not least, the perspiration which results from exercise helps wash away toxic substances, many of which may have come to roost in your joints!

Here are the morning and evening exercises frequently recommended in the readings.

MORNING WAKE-UP

A good exercise for the morning is to stand straight and tall, preferably in front of an open window (if the air outside is fresh and clean). Gradually rise up on your tiptoes, inhaling slowly and deeply, and gently bring your arms upward over your head. Then, still on your tiptoes, bend forward and bring your fingertips as far down as you are able to touch your toes. Just as your hands approach the floor, exhale in a single, forceful breath. If you are just beginning this exercise routine, repeat this exercise three times. If you feel that you can comfortably do more, work up to ten repetitions.

This stretching exercise is particularly good at giving your respiratory system a morning wake-up. An added bonus is that the tightening of leg muscles and employment of the diaphragm are particularly effective in moving the lymph, which has slowed down a great deal during your night's rest. Most important, it is a "low-impact" exercise—gentle on your joints!

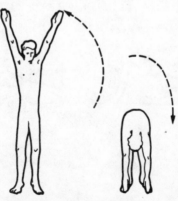

PELVIC ROLL

A specific evening exercise often recommended is the Pelvic Roll. Since it primarily exercises your lower body, it is excellent for the evening. Position yourself on the floor, face down, as if preparing to do a pushup, but place your feet flush against a wall. Raise yourself up on your arms, then rotate your hips in a circle—three times clockwise, three times counterclockwise. If you find this position too strenuous, you may actually rest on your elbows rather than your hands when assuming the pushup position.

Cayce indicated that this exercise, which rotates the lower portions of the body, would help alter circulation in a way that aided in better assimilation and elimination—which you now know to be important in preventing arthritis!

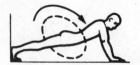 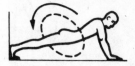

HEAD AND NECK

A unique exercise for the head and neck was mentioned in the Cayce readings over 300 hundred times. Sit with your spine erect and your shoulders relaxed. Bend your head forward three times, backward three times, to the right three times, to the left three times. Then, gently rotate your head 360 degrees in both directions three times. Do this series slowly and deliberately.

This exercise brings more circulation to the head and neck. Improved eyesight, more acute hearing, and greater relaxation are but a few of the many benefits of this routine.

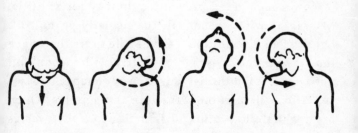

A POWERFUL PREVENTER

In hundreds of readings given for various diseases, Cayce stressed the importance of iodine in stimulating the glandular system so that it could effectively resist adverse influences. He indicated that it not only had curative but also preventative properties. Plain iodine, however, can be toxic. Because of this, Cayce usually recommended Atomidine as a supplement, which would be both safer and helpful. Taken in small doses, this substance stimulates the glands and helps bring about health. He always recommended that it be taken in cycles. Refer to Chapter Five for specific instructions on a basic routine for taking this substance.

A SPECIAL TREAT

Another excellent stimulant for the skin and the eliminations in general is massage. It is the most often recommended preventive therapy for arthritis. Massaging with special oils, particularly peanut oil, helps nurture your joints. Cayce said more than once that those who massage regularly with peanut oil need never fear arthritis! This form of therapy increases superficial circulation in the skin and muscles, which can facilitate loosening toxic buildup so that wastes can be eliminated. Seek out a local massage therapist who can provide you with both a steam and massage to receive the optimum benefits, or refer to Chapter Five for directions on self-massage.

A FINAL WORD

As you think about all the preventative therapies and health patterns above, consider one more. Regular spinal adjustments will work wonders for your health. The benefits are numerous. A good adjustment will relax you, break up toxic forces in your body, stimulate your glandular system, and nurture the proper functioning of your nervous system.

Find a good osteopath or chiropractor with whom you are comfortable. Work with him or her to devise a routine of therapy that works for you. Then stick with it. More than likely the benefits will be noticeable early on, so staying with the program will make sense to you. If you suspect you are developing arthritis, be sure to discuss it with your health-care provider. You'll be glad you did.

Chapter 5

THERAPIES MADE EASY

HOW TO USE THESE THERAPIES

The following therapies, listed in alphabetical order for easy reference, are those most often recommended by Cayce as helpful to arthritis sufferers and those in need of balancing their body systems. This chapter serves as a quick reference to help you administer the therapies suggested throughout this book.

ATOMIDINE

Atomidine was recommended time and again for arthritic patients. An iodine compound, Atomidine helps to stimulate the glands. From a physical point of view, your glands regulate your body's metabolic processes. From a spiritual point of view, the endocrine glands are the contact points between the perfect spiritual body and the physical body. Proper glandular functioning is, then, vital to your health and well-being.

Since the readings were so individualized, there are several recommended "cycles" for taking Atomidine. Here is one basic routine which is a good starting point: Take 1 drop in a half glass of water daily for 5 days, then leave off for 5 days. Repeat another one or two cycles, then leave off for a month or longer. In the mornings, before breakfast, was the suggested time of day for the dose. Specific Atomidine cycles for osteoarthritis and rheumatoid arthritis are given in the next chapter.

Notice how your body responds to this treatment, and keep up the cycles as long as you find them helpful.

Visualization Suggestion: While you drink the water containing the Atomidine, visualize the iodine entering your body and stimulating your glandular organs. Picture these systems, especially the endocrine glands (which you can look up in any anatomy book), as healthy, whole, and functioning properly. Focus on how they send out healing signals to your body.

CASTOR OIL PACKS

The purpose of castor oil packs is to stimulate the liver, colon, and the rest of the digestive tract, enhancing both assimilation and elimination. A good routine to follow for this therapy is to apply the pack three consecutive days weekly for two to three

53

weeks. Then leave off a week, and resume with another two- to three-week cycle.

For preparing and applying a pack, gather these items:

Cold-pressed castor oil

2' square of wool flannel

Large towel

2 safety pins

Small plastic trash bag

Electric heating pad

Glass or ceramic bowl

Glass jar or plastic container

2 tsp. baking soda added to a container with 1 quart of warm water

Pour heated castor oil into glass or ceramic bowl. Fold the flannel cloth to a 1' square. Place it in the bowl, saturating it with the oil, then wring out the excess. Now place the pack on the right side of your abdomen, positioned slightly toward the pelvic/liver area. Cover the pack with the plastic bag, put the heating pad on top of it, and place a towel on top of these layers, wrapping it around the body and fastening it with safety pins. Then, turn on the heating pad. You may want to lie on a plastic bag or towel to protect your bedsheets.

A good routine is to apply the pack for one-hour periods in the evening three days in a row each week for three weeks. Leave off a week, and repeat the three-day/three-week cycle, using the same days of the week and times as before. (Women should not apply the pack during their menstrual cycle.) Store the pack in a glass jar or plastic container. Packs may be reused any number of times, but should not be used by another individual.

Dip a rag into the warm water with the baking soda and clean the abdomen. The oil will contain toxins brought out through the skin and, if the abdomen is not properly cleansed, these toxins will be reabsorbed.

Visualization Suggestion: While you rest with the pack on your abdomen, imagine the increase in the releasing of toxic elements through your elimination system. Follow this with a picture of the healing oil penetrating your skin and nurturing your liver and digestive tract, bringing about a balance in the energies between your kidneys and liver.

COLONICS/ENEMAS

Stimulation of the elimination system was frequently mentioned in cases of arthritis. To help with this, enemas and colonics were occasionally recommended.

Optimally, find a therapist who can administer colonic professionally. As with spinal adjustments, you and your therapist can work out a routine that makes sense for you. Some specific colonic routines for osteoarthritis and rheumatoid arthritis are mentioned in the next chapter.

However, if you can't find a therapist, a self-administered enema will also be helpful. Here are some basic guidelines for a home enema. First, gather the following items:

Enema bag

Vaseline

Isopropyl alcohol

Pure spring water

Two large towels

Plastic trash bag

Salt

Glyco-Thymoline

Sodium bicarbonate

Begin by sterilizing with the alcohol the tube or nozzle attached to the enema bag. Prepare a quart of lukewarm spring water (98.6° F.), adding a teaspoon each of sodium bicarbonate and salt. Spread out a large plastic trash bag beneath several towels on the bed or floor and lie down in your left side. Have the bag elevated above the level of your body. Coat the enema nozzle with Vaseline and insert it two to four inches into your rectum. (Caution: Do not force it.) Allow one-third of the water to enter your colon slowly. If you begin to cramp, clamp the tube shut and take several deep breaths. Then continue. Once one-third of the water is inside, turn over on your back and allow the next third to enter, following the same procedure. Finally, shift to your right side and empty the remaining fluid from the bag into your body.

Now, try to hold the solution for five to fifteen minutes, moving gently to swish the fluid around in the colon. This allows the fluid to soften and loosen the wastes. Your next step is to use the bathroom, where you can now expel the water.

Rest a few moments, then repeat the process until the fluid which leaves your body is mostly clear. Administer a final round of water, adding a teaspoon of Glyco-Thymoline (which you can find in your health food store) to the water (instead of the salt and soda) to serve as an antiseptic to the colon area.

Visualization Suggestion: As you are experiencing the internal cleansing from a colonic or enema, picture the water rinsing and soothing your colon. As the water is expelled, imagine it carrying away toxic substances, leaving behind a clean and healthy colon. Imagine how the newly cleansed lining of your colon allows it to function better which, in turn, brings health and healing to your body.

EPSOM SALTS BATHS

An Epsom salts bath is an important therapy both in the treatment of arthritis and in the alleviation of arthritic pain.

Gather the following items to begin the bath:
4-lb. box of Epsom salts
Full tub of hot water (typically 20 gallons)
Wash cloth soaked in cool water

To administer this therapy, be sure that a friend, family member, or therapist is with you. As with all therapies, if you have heart or circulatory problems or other health considerations, such as pregnancy, consult a physician before embarking upon this treatment.

Fill tub with hot water (at a temperature you are comfortable with) and enough Epsom salts to saturate the water with the salts (usually the entire box). You'll know you've succeeded when the salts will no longer dissolve and thus settle on the bottom of the tub.

Relax in the tub for twenty to thirty minutes, with a cool cloth on your forehead. If the water begins to feel too cool, gradually increase the temperature by adding hot water. Stay in the tub for as long as you are comfortable, being sure that your body is perspiring before you complete the bath. In the case of rheumatoid arthritis, the readings often suggested that a massage be given while taking an Epsom salts bath.

Visualization Suggestion: As you relax in the tub, visualize your body's elimination system being stimulated, expelling toxic substances through your skin and lungs. As you see the wastes moving freely from your body, imagine your circulation becoming stronger and delivering nutrients to every cell of your body. Visualize yourself rising up out of the tub without pain, getting comfortably in bed, and relaxing.

EPSOM SALTS PACK

Epsom salts can also be used in pack form, administered to painful muscles and joints as often as once every day. These packs can also be helpful in relaxing the spinal area just prior to an adjustment.

For your pack, gather the following items:

1–2 cups of Epsom salts
2 gallons of very hot water
Standard size bath towel
Plastic trash bag (optional)
Heating pad (optional)

Saturate Epsom salts in very hot water. The water is considered saturated when no more salts will dissolve, thus settling on the bottom of the sink or tub. Soak the towel in the water, and apply it as hot as possible to the area to be treated. Feel free to continue re-dipping the towel in the hot water to freshen it when it cools. Application of the pack can continue for up to 2-3 hours.

One variation on this therapy is to initially prepare the towel as directed above and wrap it on the affected area. Then, cover it with the plastic and place a heating pad on top of the plastic. This way, the pack remains warm and you can relax more during the therapy.

Visualization Suggestion: As you rest, visualize the heat and Epsom salts relaxing the area on which you are concentrating. Picture the circulation building in the area, delivering nutrients to the cells which form the tissue, bone, and cartilage and carrying away toxins which have been released. See yourself resting comfortably during and after the application of the pack. Feel how good it is to have the pain released and replaced by comfort.

MASSAGE

Naturally, if you suffer severe arthritic pain, you will want a therapist to administer your massages. However, if your pain is minor, self-massage will not only be helpful but also relieving. Over 60% of the Cayce readings on arthritis recommended massage as a major preventative and therapeutic treatment.

There is a very important difference, however, in the way a massage should be given for prevention of arthritis and the way it should be given as a healing therapy to an arthritic. This difference has to do with the direction of the massage strokes. For prevention, massage strokes should be *toward the trunk of the body and the heart.* For curative therapy, massage strokes should be *away from the trunk of the body and the heart—toward the limbs.* You'll want to keep this difference in mind if you elect to do the following self-massage or discuss it with your massage therapist if you choose that route.

Below are some recommended oils, basic guidelines, and a suggested self-massage routine:

OILS FOR MASSAGE

1) Peanut oil. An excellent oil for massage, it is particularly beneficial for nerves, muscles, skin, and joints. In a few of Cayce's readings, it was strongly recommended for the prevention of arthritis. One reading went so far as to state that "Those who would take a peanut oil rub each week need never fear arthritis." (1158-31)

2) Equal parts of olive oil and peanut oil. Olive oil is particularly good for the muscles and stimulates the body's mucous-membrane activity. Mixed with an equal amount of peanut oil, this is an excellent rub for general body maintenance and arthritic pain relief.

3) Here's a more complex oil mixture which will help stimulate body energies:

Mineral oil	4 oz.
Oil of pine needles	1 oz.
Olive oil	1 oz.
Peanut oil	1 oz.
Lanolin, liquified	1 oz.

4) Finally, the following oil mixture was given to one individual as a help in the therapeutic regimen suggested for rheumatoid arthritis:

Mineral oil	4 oz.
Peanut oil	2 oz.
Sassafras root oil	1/2 oz.
Oil of pine needles	1/2 oz.
Oil of mustard	1/4 oz.

GENERAL GUIDELINES

1) For a preventative massage, strokes should be toward the heart when working on and below your shoulders. Begin with the part of the limb closest to the heart (i. e., stroke the elbow to the shoulder first; then the wrist to the elbow second; the hand third).

For a curative massage, strokes should be away

from the heart and toward the ends of the limbs, when you are working on and below your shoulders. Begin with the part of the limb closest to the trunk or heart (i.e., stroke the shoulder to the elbow first; then the elbow to the wrist second; the hand third).

2) Massage your neck and head with circular motions, trying to move the soft tissue and the skin together. In other words, do not just move your fingers on the skin.

3) Begin your strokes gently, increasing your pressure with each succeeding stroke. Then, lighten up and end with a smooth and soothing stroke. Relative to the pressure of any given stroke, your touch in massage should always be firmer toward the heart and lighter away from the heart.

4) A slower tempo will relax you, but a faster tempo will invigorate you. Choose a rhythm appropriate to your particular needs.

SUGGESTED ROUTINE FOR PREVENTATIVE MASSAGE

1) Left arm (elbow to shoulder; circular motions around elbow; wrist to elbow; knead hand; finish with a stroke of the whole arm upward, then lightly downward).

2) Right arm (follow the same directions as left arm).

3) Gently massage your abdomen, waist, and sides in an upward circular motion—your right hand moving counterclockwise (as you look down), your left hand clockwise (as you look down).

4) Left leg (knee to buttocks; circular motions around knee; ankle to knee; knead feet; finish with a stroke of the whole leg upward, then lightly downward).

5) Face (gentle, circular, upward motions).

6) Neck and shoulders (circular, kneading motions).

7) Head (circular motions moving the scalp over the skull).

SUGGESTED ROUTINE FOR CURATIVE MASSAGE

1) Left arm (shoulder to elbow; circular motions around elbow; elbow to wrist; knead hand; finish with a stroke of the whole arm downward).

2) Right arm (follow the same directions as left arm).

3) Gently massage your abdomen, waist, and sides in an upward circular motion—your right hand moving counterclockwise (as you look down), your left hand clockwise (as you look down).

4) Left leg (buttocks to knee; circular motions around knee; knee to ankle; knead feet; finish with a stroke of the whole leg downward).

5) Face (gentle, circular, upward motions).

6) Neck and shoulders (circular, kneading motions).

7) Head (circular motions moving the scalp over the skull).

Visualization Suggestion: As you massage yourself or receive a massage, visualize the strokes releasing toxic substances and sending them on their way to your elimination systems. As this free flow begins to occur, you'll feel more and more relaxed. Then picture your body absorbing the healing oils, which are nurturing your joints—all the way down to the individual cells.

OSTEOPATHIC/CHIROPRACTIC ADJUSTMENTS

The spinal column and its various counterparts are among the most mysterious and complex of your body's systems. They serve as a relay network for the life-giving signals which keep your body functioning—we hope in optimum health. Muscle tensions and spasms brought on by internal stress or external injury can decrease the movement of the vertebrae. When this happens, your general health and well-being are at risk. Manual adjustment of your spine and vertebrae is the best insurance that this important network of nerve impulses remains in good working order.

Visualization Suggestion: When receiving an osteopathic or chiropractic adjustment, visualize the flow of nerve impulses throughout your spine. See the outer reaches of your body being "fine-tuned" and these impulses stimulating healthy cellular regeneration in your joints. Remember the suggestion earlier to refer to a good anatomy book in your local library to help you develop a strong visual picture of your spine and nervous system. After the treatment, release the visual picture and enjoy the relaxed feeling of your body.

STEAMS

Here are the directions for setting up a homemade steam cabinet. Begin by gathering the following items:

Straight-backed wooden chair

Two towels

Hot plate

Pan of boiling water

Ingredient for steam additive
   (options cited below)

Old sheet

Thermometer

Pie rack

Custard cup

Find a straight-backed chair, preferably wooden, which will not be damaged by short-term heat and moisture. Drape the chair in towels so that you won't burn your body. Place a hot plate and pan of boiling water beneath the chair. Find an old sheet that you'll use as your "steam sheet" again and again. Cut a hole in the middle of the sheet large enough to fit your head through.

Just prior to your steam, drink three glasses of water. Now, undress and sit on the chair, draping the sheet around you like a tent. Be sure that the sheet does not come in contact with the hot plate. Wrap a towel around your neck to keep the steam from escaping.

For safety's sake, have a friend or family member nearby who can check on you and provide you with drinking water to keep your body fluids balanced and to increase perspiration. Be sure to check your pulse and temperature periodically. Your pulse rate should remain below 140 beats per minute (below 120 beats if you have a cardiac condition) and your temperature below 104°F.

When you have worked up a good sweat, stand up slowly, check to see that you're not feeling faint, and proceed to the bathroom. Take a cleansing shower, and afterward rub your body firmly with peanut oil, massaging your muscles and joints with deep, even strokes.

You may also wish to add special healing substances and oils to the steam process to aid in helping stimulate eliminations.

Find a small ovenproof glass dish or ceramic container (like a custard cup) and add a teaspoon of your choice of healing ingredient (only one type in any given steam). Float this cup in the pan of boiling water or place it on the pie rack above the water. The substance will vaporize as a result of the heat and help stimulate the skin.

Common additives are Atomidine, witch hazel, pine oil, wintergreen, lavender, tincture of myrrh, benzoin, and eucalyptus oil.

Visualization Suggestion: While you are enjoying your steam, feel how the increase in circulation helps break up toxic substances throughout your body, including your joints. Imagine also the positive nutrition your circulation delivers to every cell of your body.

WET-CELL APPLIANCE

The Wet-Cell Appliance or Battery is mentioned in the Cayce readings as a treatment for specific illnesses—especially those involving the nervous system and glands. It was among the most frequently mentioned and unique therapies for rheumatoid arthritis, often used following an Epsom salts bath. As Cayce described the device, it worked by awakening the autonomic nervous system or subconscious mind to help supply the body with a particular healing element. Here's a simple analogy to help us understand this process. When we watch another person eat, gastric juices are released. Our conscious mind interprets this as hunger, and we are open to the intake of food—often the food we're observing being eaten! Cayce indicated that the Wet-Cell Appliance works in the same way. The electrical current carries vibrations of the healing element which awakens in the subconscious mind the need and *receptivity* for the element. Thus, the element is invisibly assimilated into the body.

This device generates a DC current weaker than that produced by a typical D battery. The weaker current seems to imitate the natural "electrical conditions" in the body and minimize the possibility of side effects. An important part of this battery is a jar which holds a solution containing a particular healing agent. In the case of arthritis a solution of gold chloride was indicated for the jar. A low current passes through lead loops which are run through the solution. According to the readings, the electrical current picks up on a vibratory level the energy of the solution and relays it to the body.

The benefit of assimilating gold in this non-intrusive way may hold great promise for arthritis sufferers. Whereas gold treatments have helped many patients, they can also have negative side effects, such as liver and kidney damage, skin problems, and nervous disorders. This innovative therapy deserves attention and consideration because it may allow the gold to enter the body on a vibrational level, which would make it much less toxic than if it entered by injections.

Sound unbelievable? Think of it this way. Though Cayce gave these readings over 50 years ago, he was basically talking about "vibrational medicine"— a field of medical research considered to have great promise for the coming decade and millennium!

The Wet-Cell Appliance itself is actually a crude battery constructed of metal poles in a solution of sulfuric acid, copper sulfate, zinc, willow charcoal, and distilled water. The following diagram will orient you to the appliance:

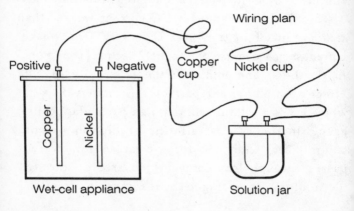

See Appendix C for the address where you can obtain more information about this device.

Visualization Suggestion: As you begin your application of the Wet-Cell, visualize your body receiving the gold chloride from the solution jar. The readings indicate that the gold will help stimulate the glands to enable the body to renew itself and release toxic forces within the system. So, visualize this happening! Concentrate on your joints, seeing them washed clean and being renewed.

Chapter 6

ROUTINES FOR RELIEF

CONSULT WITH YOUR PHYSICIAN

As with all medical problems, it is important for you to consult with your physician before you undertake any new therapies aimed at relieving your condition. Arthritis is no exception. Be sure to discuss your course of action with your physician before beginning. His or her wisdom will help you make the right decisions about your health.

PERSISTENCY AND CONSISTENCY

Two specific therapeutic regimes (see below) require persistency and consistency on your part. Don't be discouraged. There are rewards for those who harness their inner strength to make the changes in their lives that usher in healing.

RHEUMATOID ARTHRITIS

The suggested therapeutic routine outlined below is designed for those suffering from severe rheumatoid arthritis. As you work with these guidelines, you may choose to alter them according to your own condition and response.

Diet. Diet is especially important to those who suffer with rheumatoid arthritis. You should follow the recommendations regarding the acid/alkaline properties of diet and the guidelines for food combining. Also, be sure to include your six to eight glasses of water.

The following foods, listed in order of greatest helpfulness to your condition, should be part of your diet:

Carrots
Raw vegetables
Lettuce
Celery
Watercress
Green leafy vegetables
Beets
Onions
Seafood
Fish
Lamb
Fowl
Wild game

Gelatin

Cabbage

Vegetable juice

Radish

Watercress juice

V-8 juice

Yeast in V-8 juice

Beef juice

While being sure to include the above foods, avoid those listed below:

Fried foods	White potatoes
Starches	Red meat
Vinegar	Raw apples
Pork	Carbonated water

Colonics/Enemas. A colonic or high enema should be taken at the very beginning of your therapy and continued every ten days for a minimum of two months.

Osteopathic Adjustments. During your therapeutic cycle, have an osteopathic adjustment twice weekly for several weeks. Then, work with your osteopath or chiropractor to establish a continuing cycle that will be helpful to your condition.

Atomidine. Atomidine should also be a part of your therapy from the very beginning. This substance was often recommended to help correct the glandular disfunction which was playing a role in the onset of rheumatoid arthritis. Here's a routine which you can follow. Each of the suggested doses should be taken in the morning in a half glass of water.

Day 1   1 drop
Day 2   2 drops
Day 3   3 drops
Day 4   2 drops
Day 5   1 drop

Repeat this five-day cycle once every 28 days.

Epsom Salts Bath.   After the Atomidine, an Epsom salts bath should be taken. It will help break up the gradual increase of toxins at the injured sites. While you are soaking in the bath, massage or have massaged the affected limbs. An alternative to a bath is to apply Epsom salts packs to the specific areas.

Massage.   After the Epsom salts bath, a full-body massage should be taken using pure peanut oil. This will help your body take full advantage of the therapeutic effects of the Epsom salts bath and the massage. Continue having a massage each day for two weeks using the pure peanut oil.

Wet-Cell Battery.   The Wet-Cell Battery can be used in conjunction with this cycle of therapies, also after the Epsom salts bath. Three grains of gold chloride to three ounces of water should be used in the solution jar. According to the readings, gold could have a positive effect upon the rejuvenation of the glands. In the case of rheumatoid arthritis, the readings suggested that the Wet-Cell be charged with iodine. Directions for this procedure can be obtained from the supplier.

Continue Therapy. After two weeks of massage and rest, repeat the cycle, beginning with the Atomidine routine.

OSTEOARTHRITIS

The following therapeutic routine provides a suggested course of action for beginning to apply the Cayce readings' ideas to your arthritic condition. They are particularly tailored for osteoarthritis sufferers, but may also be helpful to those with mild cases of rheumatoid arthritis. As you work with these ideas, it is important to listen to your body, making adjustments that you feel are helpful to your particular condition.

Diet. Your diet should follow the recommendations regarding the acid/alkaline properties of food as well as the guidelines for food combining. Also, remember to drink six to eight glasses of water a day. As you design your diet, be sure to include a variety of the following foods:

Fish	Fowl
Lamb	Raw vegetables
Citrus fruit juices	Carrots
Fruit	Beef juice
Steamed vegetables	Wild game
Seafood	Beets
Leafy vegetables	Gelatin
Liver	Green vegetables

Celery	Lettuce
Whole grain cereal	Egg yolk
Vegetable juices	Watercress
Whole wheat bread	Jerusalem artichokes
Carrot juice	Vegetable soup
Nuts	Figs

While being sure to include the above foods, avoid those listed below:

Fried foods	White potatoes
Starches	Red meat
Vinegar	Raw apples
Pork	Carbonated water

Colonics/Enemas. If you suspect that your eliminations are less than optimum, take the time before you begin other therapies to have a series of two to three enemas, four days apart.

Atomidine. As with rheumatoid arthritis, Atomidine should also be a part of your therapy from the very beginning. Here's a routine which you can follow. Each of the suggested doses should be taken in the morning in a half glass of water.

Day 1	1 drop
Day 2	2 drops
Day 3	3 drops
Day 4	2 drops
Day 5	1 drop

Repeat this five-day cycle once every 28 days.

Epsom Salts Bath. When you complete the series of Atomidine drops, take an Epsom salts bath.

While in the bath, massage or have massaged the joints affected.

Massage. When you finish the above Epsom salts bath, have a full-body massage with an oil mixture of half peanut oil, half olive oil. Pay particular attention to the affected joints. For the following two weeks, have a massage every other night.

Continue Therapy. Repeat the above cycle of therapy, beginning with the five-day cycle of Atomidine through the two weeks of massage.

GENTLE REMINDER

The above therapies are meant as guidelines for you to use in your discussion with your physician. As you work with them, listen to what your body is telling you. Somewhere deep inside it is trying to give you hints as to what you need to do to bring about healing. Be sure to listen—and respond!

CONCLUSION

As you work with the ideas in this book, you'll begin to develop a closer bond with your body. It is important that you grow to love and respect every inch of it, from head to toe. This includes even the parts of you that give you aches and pains. A sore and swollen joint is a part of the special gift you received when you were born. Begin by nurturing these feelings of thankfulness, and the spirit within will respond more readily with healing energies. Remember your purpose: to be healed that you might serve others!

Once you feel that flow of nurturance, focus it on the task at hand. Remember to imagine positive events happening, on a physical level, as you practice the therapies in this book. Whether you are working on improving your eliminations, eating the right foods, or even relaxing in a hot bath, visualize success. The simple act of visualization may be the component that some of your past efforts lacked. Finally, remember to be consistent and persistent in your efforts. Don't give up if you have a bad day. Simply smile and believe that tomorrow will be better. If you stay on the road to health, taking as few detours as possible, your destination can be realized.

This, of course, brings us back to a point we discussed earlier in the book—*hope*. Perhaps one of the overlooked "medicines" which packs the greatest power is the ability of the human spirit to hope. This quality of spirit can have a tremendous effect on the physical, if we allow it.

Best wishes for better health and happiness!

APPENDIX A

WHO WAS EDGAR CAYCE?

Edgar Cayce exhibited unusual psychic ability at an early age and soon became known for his remarkable clairvoyant gifts. In a self-induced hypnotic state, he was able to diagnose illnesses and prescribe remedies with remarkable success. Often referred to as "the sleeping prophet" and the world's most documented psychic, Edgar Cayce left behind a legacy of over 14,000 psychic readings covering such subjects as healing, dreams, meditation, reincarnation, prophecy, and psychic ability.

Born in 1877 in Hopkinsville, Kentucky, he discovered by accident that he could absorb information on any particular subject merely by napping for a while on a book pertaining to that topic. At the age of fifteen he suffered an accident, and, while in a coma, instructed his astonished parents to prepare a poultice to be applied at the base of his brain. The application fully restored him.

After he reached adulthood, his job as a salesman was threatened by a mysterious paralysis of the throat muscles which medical doctors were unable to treat. He consulted a hypnotist, and it was under the subsequent trance that Edgar correctly diagnosed his condition and prescribed an almost immediate cure.

Not long after, Edgar discovered that his gift could be used to help others, and what followed was over forty years of helping people from his self-induced state of unconsciousness. For twenty-two of these years, his readings were largely confined to medical problems; however, the scope of Edgar's abilities expanded in later years to include such subjects as meditation, dreams, reincarnation, and the Bible.

Edgar Cayce is regarded today as one of the most significant explorers of the human psyche in the twentieth century.

APPENDIX B

HOW THE A.R.E. CAN HELP YOU

A wealth of information from the Edgar Cayce readings is available to you on hundreds of topics, from astrology and arthritis to universal laws and world affairs, through the organization which Edgar Cayce founded in 1931, the Association for Research and Enlightenment, Inc.

The facilities and benefits offered by the A.R.E. include the largest body of documented psychic information anywhere in the world: the 14,263 Cayce readings, copies of which are housed in the A.R.E. Library/Conference Center in Virginia Beach, Virginia. These readings have been indexed under 10,000 different topics and are currently being placed on computer. They are available to the public.

Membership in the A.R.E. is inexpensive and includes benefits such as: the bimonthly magazine, *Venture Inward;* home-study lessons in spiritual awareness and growth; the A.R.E. Library, available to you through book-borrowing by mail, offering collections of the actual Edgar Cayce readings as well as access to one of the world's best parapsychological book collections; and the names of medical doctors or health care professionals in your area who are willing to work with the remedies prescribed in the Edgar Cayce readings.

As an organization on the leading edge of exciting new fields of study, A.R.E. also presents seminars around the nation, led by prominent authorities in various fields and exploring such areas as parapsychology, dreams, meditation, personal growth, world religions, reincarnation and life after death, and holistic health.

The unique path to personal growth outlined in the Cayce readings is developed through a worldwide program of study groups. These informal groups meet weekly in private homes—right in your community—for friendly consciousness-expanding discussions.

A.R.E. maintains a visitors' center that offers a well-stocked bookstore, exhibits, classes, a movie, and audiovisual presentations to introduce seekers from all walks of life to the fascinating concepts found in the Cayce readings.

A.R.E. conducts ongoing research into the helpfulness of both the medical and nonmedical readings, often giving members the opportunity to participate in the studies themselves.

For more information and a free color brochure, write or phone:

A.R.E.

P.O. Box 595

67th Street and Atlantic Avenue

Virginia Beach, VA 23451-0595, (804) 428-3588

APPENDIX C

WHERE TO FIND THE
REMEDIES AND INGREDIENTS

Some of the formulations mentioned in the Edgar
Cayce readings are available from:

Home Health Products
P.O. Box 3130
Virginia Beach, VA 23454

Information about the Wet-Cell Appliance is available
from:

The A.R.E. Clinic
4018 N. 40th St.
Phoenix, AZ 85018